The True Story of Sam: Some Things All Bicyclists Should Know

Samuel E. Shull

authorHOUSE®

About the Author

The author was an avid bicyclist and a very competitive bicycle racer for many years. He is a retired engineer holding an A.B. degree from Franklin and Marshall College and B.S., M.S. degrees in Chemical Engineering from the University of Pennsylvania. His career path was in the chemical industry where he held a wide variety of staff and management positions serving R&D and Engineering functions.

AuthorHouse™
1663 Liberty Drive
Bloomington, IN 47403
www.authorhouse.com
Phone: 1-800-839-8640

The material contained in this book is for information purposes only. No medical therapy or exercise program should be undertaken except under the direction of a physician. Mention of specific products or companies does not imply endorsement by the author. The author and publisher of this text make no warranties, expressed or implied, about the value for any purpose of the information and ideas contained herein.

Published by AuthorHouse   06/05/2012

ISBN: 978-1-4772-1640-8 (sc)
ISBN: 978-1-4772-1639-2 (e)

Library of Congress Control Number: 2012910296

This book is printed on acid-free paper.

DEDICATION

To my loving wife Lois who has followed my interest and involvement in bicycling for over forty years. I thank her for her support, even though at times we did not always agree that my biking-related pursuits were headed in the right direction. Lois was instrumental in helping with the preparation and review of this text.

ACKNOWLEDGMENT

I will be forever grateful to Stanley J. Antolak, Jr., M.D. in Coon Rapids, Minnesota. He was the only doctor of many I had seen who, about six years ago, was able to diagnose and treat the extreme pain in my buttocks whenever I sat down. The problem was related to my pudendal nerve. To me Dr. Antolak is the leading authority regarding the diagnosis, differentiation, and treatment of pudendal neuralgia versus other forms of pelvic pain such as prostatitis. He has made and continues to make presentations throughout the world trying to educate the medical profession in a field of technology where there is extremely limited expertise. Dr. Antolak is founder and director of the Center for Urologic and Pelvic Pain which is now a part of the Medical Advanced Pain Clinics (MAPS) in Coon Rapids, Minnesota.

Many thanks to my urologist, Anita H. Tekchandani, M.D. who provided me with a firm diagnosis of interstitial cystitis (IC) as a reason for my pelvic pain and general guidelines for managing such.

Special thanks to my rehabilitation doctor Leslie H. Schutz, M.D. who provided me with specific details regarding injury to my lumbar spine and a specific framework of stretching and strengthening exercises so that I could resume doing some of the things in life which I most enjoy. Initially Dr. Schutz was my biggest motivator. When she told me that my goals for self-improvement were too lofty, I looked for ways to upgrade my stretching and strength-building program. She was the one who really motivated me to search hard for other means which might be applicable to help address the downside of the aging process.

Our older son Richard did the most to build my interest in cycling. Over many years, his interest and enthusiasm for cycling continued to rub off on me. He has wonderful mechanical ability and was always most helpful in servicing my bikes. Often we would time trial against one another in the hills of rural Pennsylvania, and I had to continually negotiate for larger and larger handicaps. One day, which I will never forget, he had given me a handicap of twelve minutes. I had just climbed up one large hill and was heading down the second at a speed of about 35 MPH in front of a farm house when a large rooster came up from a roadside gulley and crossed right in front of me. I hit the rooster head-on and flew over the handlebars, landing at the side of the roadway. I was very badly bruised but fortunately had no broken bones. I will be forever thankful that I was wearing a good bicycle helmet. My son showed up about five minutes after the incident and helped get me home. Thank you, Richard! We looked for signs of the rooster, but could find none – only a couple small feathers in my chain.

Thanks to my new personal physician, Jakub Malarz, M.D. Dr. Malarz provided me with a hyaluronic acid based gel which was extremely effective in eradicating a host of facial blemishes. I was hopeful that this might be a stepping stone to the use of oral HA supplements for better skin, joint and eye health, but such was contraindicated.

FOREWARD

I have written this book so that others within and outside the cycling community might benefit from my biking experience, including details as to how I have successfully managed recovery from very serious injury. By writing this book detailing my experience, I believe I have found a unique opportunity to provide meaningful "give back" for benefits derived from over 50 years of bicycling and bicycle racing. As a result of information summarized in the text, I believe the potential exists for many readers to find a better quality of life and avoid horrendous pain and distress. Only in my later years did I realize that vigorous cycling might have a cumulative potential to precipitate such serious injury and many health-related problems. I discuss in this book in some detail the injury to my pudendal nerve, which terminated my biking and competitive racing career at age 70. Related injuries (interstitial cystitis and low back) are also addressed.

As part of a six-year recovery process, I have had the opportunity to research and evaluate diet and other parameters which relate to inflammation. Such have opened up a second story line which is addressed in the text regarding related improvements in my health.

This book is for informational purposes only. One should not try any of my medical/rehabilitation adventures without first checking with their doctor.

PREFACE

Over the years I have had a passion for bicycling and bicycle racing. Such was forever terminated about six years ago when I could not sit in the car for a ten-minute drive to the grocery store because of extreme pain in the buttocks. This problem was ultimately characterized as pudendal neuralgia. Within the next year or two, a related nerve and bladder problem, interstitial cystitis (IC) developed. New problems developed with the lower back and became so painful that I had trouble swinging a golf club and bending over to pick up the club and golf ball. Often I could not walk more than a mile without the right knee aching and occasionally it would crack with each step. I had been knocked down and really had little hope for an essentially complete recovery.

As the result of several rather dramatic health improvements, including many which came about within the past year, I thought maybe I could race that bicycle again. Checkouts on an indoor trainer for 30 minutes at near maximum heart rate, 3 to 4 times per week for 3 months left me ready to tell the world that I could now ride a time trial bike faster than I could 15 years ago. After my wife Lois kept asking me, whenever I experienced very occasional pelvic pain, "Were you riding that bicycle again?", I reevaluated the whole situation. Perhaps she and the doctor in Minnesota who first diagnosed my nerve problem were indeed correct when they both said DO NOT RIDE THE BIKE!

This book tells my story. I believe both the cycling community and general population can benefit from my experience regarding critical health issues, all addressed in the following chapters.

God has been good to me. I intend to donate any profit which may result from the sale of this book to support miscellaneous Christian ministries, as well as the Senior Services organization in Midland, MI.

Contents

Chapter 1

About Sam

I was born in Lancaster, PA. In my youth I spent many, many hours biking the roads in rural Lancaster County. In the late 1960s I moved with my wife and family to the Williamsport, PA area where I discovered the thrill of bicycle racing. I developed a deep passion for the sport. I was introduced to the sport of racing by my son Richard, who ultimately raced with the cycling team at Cornell University in Ithaca, NY. My first real experience training with Richard in the mountains surrounding Williamsport was not a good one. I quickly "pooped out" and needed a rope tow by Richard back to our transport vehicle. I quickly learned, as a result of this event, that excellent conditioning is a prerequisite to successful bicycle racing.

For about thirty years I competed in many racing events. Such included local area races, state and national United States Cycling Federation events, state and national Senior Olympics (now called National Senior Games) and team triathlons. I always finished near the top of the competition field and never lost my passion for training or racing.

I believe my greatest cycling accomplishment was winning a 20-kilometer time trial during the 1993 National Senior Games in Baton Rouge, LA. Competition was with 65 competitors in the 55 to 60 age group from the United States, Mexico and Canada. I continued to actively pursue racing until 2005, when at the age of 70 I experienced severe pain, first in the buttocks and then later in the lower back. I describe the approach to dealing with these ailments in subsequent sections as well as my continuing motivation to set new goals for self-improvement.

2

Why Active Bicyclists and Many Others Should Have Pudendal Nerve Awareness

I am certain that 99 plus percent of you have never heard of the pudendal nerve. Neither have a very high percentage of those in the medical profession and those who have know little about it.

The pudendal nerve originates in the pelvic region. There are three branches associated with the nerve: a rectal branch, perineal branch, and clitoral/penile branch (female/male). The nerve is responsible for orgasm, urination and defecation. Its pathway may be tortuous among ligaments, muscles and other body structures, which if altered may damage the nerve. The pain associated with such damage can be horrendous. Individuals, particularly those who have no understanding of the problem and have no idea who to contact for help or how to treat it, have become suicidal. Recognizing the symptoms of potential nerve problems and taking prompt action is very important. Once the damage reaches a certain point, it may become irreversible. If nerve entrapment occurs and invasive surgery is required, chances for a "good recovery" may be remote.

2. WHY ACTIVE BICYCLISTS AND MANY OTHERS SHOULD HAVE PUDENDAL NERVE AWARENESS

It is important, but true, that the mainstream medical profession has little knowledge about pudendal neuralgia (PN). Such is defined by Taber's Cyclopedic Medical Dictionary1 as pain occurring along the course of the nerve [5]. It may be caused by pressure on nerve trunks, nutritional deficiencies, toxins or inflammation. A major symptom is pain when sitting. Frequently there are urinary, rectal or sexual problems. Individuals prone to pudendal neuralgia in addition to cyclists may be those who had chronic constipation, prior pelvic surgery, frequent infections, a hard fall, difficult childbirth or actual entrapment, each of which could remodel the nerve.

The cyclist can be particularly vulnerable to pudendal neuralgia (PN). Prolonged sitting, often with poorly padded cycling shorts on hard, narrow poorly designed and positioned saddles, coupled with repetitive movement and hard thrusting of the legs may seriously compromise the health of the nerve. In some circles, pudendal neuralgia is referred to as cyclists' syndrome. Men and women have common symptoms for pudendal neuralgia. It does not seem to significantly impact one sex more than the other. It is not age related.

The prevalence of pudendal neuralgia in this country appears to be unknown. Very frequently pudendal nerve problems are misdiagnosed as chronic non-bacterial prostatitis (five times for me by different doctors) or some other problem such as interstitial cystitis, which causes pain in the pelvic area [1]. One problem is that much understanding of pudendal nerve issues is so recent that in many cases they have gone misdiagnosed or undiagnosed for years.

I have developed pudendal neuralgia as described above and in several instances experienced the horrendous pain mentioned. In Chapters 3 and 4 I recount some of the events that terminated my bicycling career along with the doctor's assessment of my condition and prescribed treatment. However, before concluding this chapter, I want to share with you, as an addendum to this chapter, some comments from my friend Kris in Belgium. He has given me permission to include his story in the book. Kris's condition and experience is similar but not identical to mine. In his case nerve damage has

4

progressed to the point of actual entrapment (PNE). His story helps illustrate what damage to the nerve can do to one's life.

ADDENDUM: Kris' Story

I am a 47-year-old male, I work in IT involving sitting all day long, and in my free time I was a avid cyclist and runner. I often ran more than 50 km a week and cycled 250 km in one week. Everybody should say ..you are very healthy . right ?? I remember the first time I felt 'it ' was almost 7 years ago in the beginning of October 2004. I still remember the date as the feeling has never left me since then. I first felt it when getting up from a normal (hard) chair and also a few hours after another bike session .It was a strange feeling under my left buttock. A feeling I never had, .. a stabbing painful thing, cold and warm sensations. I found out, and the onset was very sudden, that I couldn't sit anymore for any time like + 15 minutes. Strange as I never had any problem at that location. The first days I thought it was a minor issue and tried to keep on cycling, but after a few miles I found out that the pain was just too bad to continue. From then on I stopped cycling completely. I also found out soon enough that I couldn't sit on a normal chair anymore, and had problems sitting in my car, So the long search (almost 3 years) began to find out what exactly was wrong. I first went to a sport doctor who operated on me for bursitis and did a hamstring release, after a lot of steroid injections. Of course the surgery didn't help as I already expected, because the top of the hamstring is about 5 cm from the place where my pain is situated. Then I tried nerve blocks which had a very temporary effect. Also heating (Rhizomy) the nerve didn't have any real result for my pain. I also went for physical therapy for almost a year but the result was... I couldn't sit!! I then found this website and did some investigations myself. I collected success and failure statistics and found out that the last option, PN decompression surgery, was risky. Especially for me, because although I couldn't sit, it was the 'only ' problem I have.

2. WHY ACTIVE BICYCLISTS AND MANY OTHERS SHOULD HAVE PUDENDAL NERVE AWARENESS

If I read this now it sounds like it wasn't so bad but it was! The pain when I sat down was so big I couldn't concentrate on my work anymore. Working became impossible and a real torture. However, most PI members have more issues and I found out were worse than I was , even if I couldn't imagine then how that would be possible as by this time I was very, very frustrated with it. As time moved on I learned that although sitting was making my pain worse over the day, it didn't make my overall pain worse either! So how strange it may sound, I became less stressed with it knowing just this. I went to Dr De Bischop in France and he also thought I had PNE. I also went to another doctor, Dr Beco in Belgium, and he confirmed that I had PNE, he recommended surgery but I thought the risk of getting worse by decompression surgery was too big for me at that time. I found out that although there are people who did get better by this surgery, some got worse. And of course the more things you are still able to, the more you have to lose I thought. Doctor Beco said to me that it was best not to sit for a long time after surgery anyway, so this didn't sound as a good way out to solve my problems anyway because of my occupation. I then found out that neuro-stimulation is another option. I also found out that this doctor was radically against release surgery so it confused me even more. I then saw Dr JP Van Buyten in Belgium and I opted for the option of neuro-stimulation, because if this doesn't work the doctors could undo it. In the meantime I kept on searching for a solution to sit at work, which was my biggest worry. I was fine when I didn't have to sit, like on every weekend. But in a normal life, most days I was shattered at 11 o'clock in the morning, because I had to work. While being on the waiting list for neuro-stimulation, I discovered that driving in a camper van was something I could do for a longer time (2 hours) without too much pain. After sitting in that for a few days without sitting on something else and of course limiting the sitting time altogether I felt usually much better. First I thought it was because of less stress or being in another environment, or so because typically the pain subsided over at least a week and a worse seat doesn't bring more pain instantly. I had tried about 15 different chairs at the office, I even tried standing for the whole day, lying down etc. I have tried Lyrica . With the pills I could sit a little longer, but I had to take so much of them that I couldn't concentrate because of the side effects of the medicine. So I investigated this car seat very carefully and found out that the shape of the top of the chair was the most important. The top was firm enough to support my weight, without leaving any pressure in the middle, which is where my pain is. A racecar chair that is a bit too small is the best description. So I bought some extra car chairs just like that and with them I built a few chairs for the office, at home and I even made them a bit better by removing some material from the middle and making the sides firmer. By the time it was my turn to try the neuro-stimulation I postponed it for 3 months and again and then cancelled it altogether. This was because I then could sit for 3 or 4 hours in a row without too much pain. Because evolution is so slow and it was a wavelike pain anyway, it took a lot of time before you could even say for sure something was happening. I can sit now for almost a full day, without too much pain. Sure I can feel it at the end of the day but it is milder than it ever was. Sitting on a 'normal' chair for an hour or so gives back the pain like before. If I stay careful on the other hand I feel that my tense and painful muscles relax as time goes on, and that alone makes the pain less. It is then less worse if I have to sit for social events and places where I cannot control the 'sitting gear' but honestly, I still try to avoid as much sitting on 'other chairs' as I possibly can. I have the feeling that over the past 2 years I am beginning to get better, very very slooowwly . I once had a pain therapist that told me that the problem would settle if I am just patient enough. When I asked him how long that would be, he responded . . . "about 10 years, because in the end your nerve will give up and not grow where the damage is." I was frustrated with this answer at the time, but now I think, that this guy could have been right. So, I think for my problem I made the best choice by not having the decompression surgery. I'm absolutely sure I got it from cycling so I would say to others . . . use those padded cycling shorts before you get it, (I never did), get a softer seat if any exists BEFORE you feel any pain ..And ....Don't overdo anything. Now I ride a recumbant bike which I can use for hours as there is no pressure on my buttocks.I use a special car (TWIKE) as most cars still bring me pain. I realize that my case differs from what many people have to endure but I also think that there is a risk of jumping into serious surgery too soon. My advice would be If there is ANY chance of getting your life back without surgery, try that first, as the surgery is certainly no picnic, and certainly also something that takes a lot of time. Kris Reference: Health Organization for Pudendal Education [http://www.pudendalhope.info/node/70]. Thank you, Kris.

3

Termination of Bicycling Career at Age 70

About five years ago I was having severe pain and burning in the buttocks. I could not even sit down in the car for a ten-minute drive to the grocery store. My wife and I had been searching unsuccessfully for several months for someone who could diagnose and treat the problem which was continuing to worsen. Finally I asked my wife to drive me 2 ½ hours to see a urologist affiliated with the University of Michigan, whom I had seen previously. His prior diagnosis was chronic non-bacterial prostatitis. He said I should go home and take two Alleve every day. I thought perhaps he could help with the pain and burning in my rear end which we never had discussed previously. He said he could not. He did suggest that I acquire and review a copy of the book A Headache in the Pelvis, by David Wise, Ph.D. and Rodney Anderson, M.D. [8] I did so and found that the book contained two paragraphs on Pudendal Nerve Entrapment (PNE). Two sentences in those two paragraphs struck me like a bolt of lightning. "Patients with this syndrome typically have considerable pain while sitting that is completely removed when standing. It is also considerably relieved by sitting on a toilet seat." I jumped out of my chair, telling my wife that the pudendal nerve absolutely must be the cause of my problem. She agreed.

I immediately began my search to find individuals who were knowledgeable about treatment of the pudendal nerve, but discovered that there was only a very small group of such people in the United States. I was looking for a doctor who would take a very conservative or self-care approach to treatment, if such were possible. Fortunately I was able to find a contact who provided me with a strong recommendation. My contact suggested that I reach Stanley J. Antolak, Jr., M.D. in Minnesota. The contact seemed confident that he could help me and do so in a timely fashion. I immediately set up an appointment with Dr. Antolak, but found that he could not see me for six weeks. In the meantime, the pain became so bad that my wife had to take me to the emergency department of the local hospital. They put me on morphine for pain control. When I told them that I was absolutely certain my problem related to the pudendal nerve, they put me on medication to control nerve pain. That worked and I was able to lead a reasonably normal life until I was able to see Dr. Antolak.

I want to jump ahead and tell the reader about some highlights regarding subjects which are detailed in subsequent chapters. A primary objective in writing this book is to point out to the reader that there may be hope and treatment for pelvic pain for which no definitive cause has been established. Such could relate to the pudendal nerve, particularly if the pain occurs in the buttocks when sitting. I can tell the reader that for pudendal neuralgia cases such as mine, rapid progress with simple treatment can occur during the first year and such can be effectively measured.

Within only a year or two after receiving a confirming PN diagnosis, I received a positive confirmation of interstitial cystitis (IC). New problems which developed with the lower back became so painful that I had trouble bending over to pick up the golf club and ball. Often I could not walk more than a mile without the right knee aching.

Recovery from all the above ailments has been remarkably positive. Details may be found in subsequent chapters. Unfortunately, however, my cycling career must be officially considered terminated at age 70.

4

Doctor's Diagnosis and Treatment - A Six-year Time Frame

About six years ago Dr. Antolak informed me that I had pudendal neuralgia (PN). I have a serious problem of pain consisting mainly of rectal burning but also distinct and bothersome suprapubic pressure. I had aggravated the nerve by excessive exercise activities, most notably cycling, over the years. They could not determine the extent or permanence of the damage. No evidence of nerve entrapment (PNE) was found. A Pudendal Nerve Motor Latency Test was normal. Some quantitative testing helped confirm the pudendal neuropathy. Pudendal neuropathy is any disease relating to the pudendal nerve or one of its branches. (The terms pudendal neuralgia and pudendal neuropathy are used interchangeably by many.) I had distinct abnormalities at several sites in the pudendal nerve distribution.

In reviewing my history, I was told that my rectal pain, aggravated by sitting and relieved by standing, recumbent, and sitting on a toilet seat was typical for pudendal neuropathy. Prior doctor visits regarding voiding problems may have been indicative of neuropathy at that time. Dr. Antolak mentioned that surgeries involving the pelvic area (and I had several) could damage the nerve. He told me that constipation will cause problems with pudendal nerve stretching and damage to the nerve. He went on to tell me that pudendal nerve damage also bothers the colon and causes constipation. Actually, I failed to tell Dr. Antolak that I had severe constipation years ago and because of it developed an anal fissure requiring two separate surgeries. In fact, it had to be redone because it failed the first time. I believe that next to cycling, constipation may have been the greatest cause of my nerve damage.

Initially my treatment involved a series of three bilateral nerve blocks performed by a neurosurgeon at four-week intervals. The most important treatment step, however, was implementation of a rigorous program of self-management care. Such is done with all Dr. Antolak's patients with pudendal neuropathy. I was prescribed medication for nerve pain which was ultimately changed to Gabapentin. I continue to use such today.

Unfortunately I had to find out through the School of Hard Knocks that every one of the following DO-NO-Dos has real meaning. Finding a quick solution to the problem is certainly important and desirable; however, one might regret the final outcome if the initial approach is not conservative. Dr. Antolak's basic pudendal neuropathy instructions were:

DO NOT SIT - DO NOT SIT - DO NOT SIT

1. Stop ALL exercises except walking on a flat surface, pushups or chinups, and swimming with a pool buoy to avoid the kick. Wear loose clothing that keeps pressure off your bottom.

2. If sitting is necessary, make a "perineal suspension pad." The concept is to sit on a pad that suspends the perineum and relieves pressure on the pudendal nerve. (I have purchased cushions from the Interstitial Cystitis Network which work very well. I currently use one with few exceptions whenever sitting. Yes, even after six years.)

Squatting
Abdominal crunches
Cycling
Leg presses
Piriformis stretches
Pilates
Gym workouts
Step aerobics
Stairmaster
Yoga
Elliptical trainer
Skiing
Exercise cycle
Jogging
Lifting
Spinning
Bowling
Stair Climbing (avoid when possible)
Sit-ups

Table 4.1: Dr. Antolak's "Do Not Do" List

3. Lie down as much as possible for TV, reading, etc. (I tried to follow this guideline in the early phase of treatment.)
4. **DO NOT DO** the listed activities on the "Do Not Do" list in Table 4.1!!

Dr. Antolak emphasized that I should try to avoid all hip flexion activities such as sitting, climbing, squatting or general exercising. Such could induce pelvic or prostatitis-like pain. Walking was okay, but I should not push the speed beyond 3.7 MPH. Okay to swim provided I used a pool buoy to avoid the kick. Golfing was okay, but I should try to avoid too much bending. Pushups and pullups were okay. Dr. Antolak told me that self-management means it is important that I do not pursue exercise activities other than these. When I asked him about riding the bike, he told me that IT WOULD PROBABLY BE BEST IF I DID NOT ATTEMPT TO RIDE THE BIKE AGAIN IN MY LIFETIME.

Recovery over a Six-year Time Frame

Recovery in large part was assessed by reviewing NIH-Chronic Prostatitis Symptoms Index Scores [CPSI]. The final score reflects a summation resulting from a detailed review of Pain and Urinary Symptoms and a Quality of Life Assessment. These surveys in general were taken quarterly but more frequently early in the treatment process.

Baseline (First Office Visit, Jan. 2007)

I had significant perineal pain, felt terrible. A CPSI score of 22.

The First year (2007)

My progress was rapid and truly amazing. In the first year I complied in virtually every way with Dr. Antolak's DO-NOT-DO instructions. Six months after the third nerve block, I had no pain in the perineum and very rarely in the pubic/bladder area. I had reduced my CPSI number to 8. I started using 300 mg/day Gabapentin instead of Tegretol for pain control. There was no discomfort whatsoever in driving an automobile. At my one-year anniversary, my pain scores were all zero, my CPSI score 3. Three months later, twelve months after the third nerve block, my pain scores were again zero. I never had any evidence of pain or discomfort in the perineum or pubic/bladder area.

The Second year (2008)

The first quarter of the second year started in the same way the first year finished. The second quarter, however, was a disaster. I was having some pubic/bladder area problems and eventually received a firm diagnosis of interstitial cystitis from my urologist. (Chapter 5 addresses the IC issue.) Within weeks of the IC diagnosis, I got "run over by a truck."

Two days before I had to run a Thursday Meals on Wheels delivery route, my IC pain continued to snowball downhill. I had been extremely careful to avoid all foods on the IC "hit list." My butt burned during the entire time of the three-hour Meals on Wheels delivery. That Friday, Saturday and all day Sunday I was in misery. By bedtime Sunday I was a basket case. I had pain in the entire pelvic area including the genitals and butt (pain front and rear). I had gone off all medications except Gabapentin at the 600 mg/day level. I told my wife that I was about ready to jump off a cliff (no, not really, but I knew from the butt pain that somehow I was severely irritating the pudendal nerve). I had to find out what to do about it and do so quickly.

After reviewing all the literature I could find on IC and hundreds of pages regarding the pudendal nerve, I decided to increase the Gabapentin dose from 600 to 1200 mg/day. Results were a dramatic reduction in both IC and perineal pain. Some time ago I had been taking no Gabapentin whatsoever. I started taking it at the 600 mg/day level when significant IC symptoms started to appear. I continued to take Gabapentin at the 1200 mg/day level.

Very significant levels of pubic/bladder area pain were experienced in the 2nd and 3rd quarters of the second year. High levels of pain correlate with high CPSI scores of 18 and 17 in the 2nd and 3rd quarters. A lower CPSI score of 8 in the 4th quarter may reflect the use of 1200 mg/day Gabapentin for pain control.

In the late 4th quarter, the formal program to help improve my back stability and reduce pain was just beginning. This program involved use of Life Fitness® Seated Row, Lat Pulldown, Leg Press,

Glute, and Elliptical trainer machines. A Gravitron/Stairmaster® pullup/dip machine was also utilized.

The Third Year (2009)

I advised Dr. Antolak that I received a confirming diagnosis of interstitial cystitis (IC) – Chapter 5. Dr. Antolak responded by telling me that he was not at all surprised. He told me that IC is a component of pudendal neuralgia with neurogenic inflammation of the bladder.

The early part of the third year was very bad. Frequent and often severe pain in the genitals and pubic/bladder area. No pain in the butt or perineum. CPSI score 25. Quality of life, mostly dissatisfied. My condition seemed to stabilize (CPSI 7) in the latter part of the year after abandoning all high intensity leg press activity. Such was incorporated into my back treatment program started at the end of the second year. I had uncertainty about use of the leg press machine but failed to flag it as being unacceptable.

In the latter part of the third year, I was pleased with quality of life (CPSI score 7). Interstitial cystitis seemed to be controlled by the use of 1200 mg/day Gabapentin and avoiding acidic foods. With perfect hindsight, I now realize it should have been at this point that I clearly understood that treatment practice for the pudendal nerve versus that for back and spine were incompatible (see Chapter 6 for further discussion). Instead I just continued to do foolish things which might permanently irritate or injure the pudendal nerve (including the bladder).

The Fourth Year (2010)

Looking back, I am almost too embarrassed to tell you how I behaved in 2010 and clung to thoughts and ideas which never should have entered my mind. On the physical side, frequent pubic/bladder area pain was my biggest problem. I failed to realize at that time that I was conforming extremely poorly to my doctor's DO-NOT-DO instructions. If I continued in such a manner, I now believe that I would never have had a chance of solving the pain problems in the pubic/bladder area and might do permanent damage to the nerve.

In the fourth year my CPSI scores were very good ranging from 3 to 8. In this time frame I rated Quality of Life at a level somewhere between mostly satisfied and delighted. Somehow this quality of life must have been sufficient to allow more foolish thoughts to creep into my small mind. For example:

- Since I recognized that I should not ride the bicycle, I decided to take up and learn the sport of race walking (most likely in itself a DO-NOT-DO). But probably worse were the DO-NOT-Dos associated with training for the sport of race walking (e.g. Piriformis stretches, and I did several of them). I competed in the Michigan Senior Olympics, did well and even qualified for the National event, but unfortunately I was at this point almost totally ignoring my doctor's DO-NOT-DO instructions.
- Motivated in part by the success in race walking, I began experimenting with easy rides on the stationary bike. This activity was my doctor's absolute DO-NOT-DO. I had a grand vision at this time of being able once again to ride a time trial bike at the competitive level.

I did not come to my senses until the end of the Fifth Year.

The Fifth Year (2011)

I was so pleased with the quality of life that I committed an unpardonable sin and may have to pay a price for it. Let me tell you about it.

As the result of several rather dramatic health improvements, including many which came about within the past year, I thought maybe I could race that bicycle again. Checkouts on an indoor trainer for 30 minutes at near maximum heart rate, 3 to 4 times per week for 3 months left me ready to tell the world that I could now ride a time trial bike faster than I could 15 years ago. After my wife Lois kept asking me, whenever I experienced that occasional pelvic pain, "Were you riding that bicycle again?, I reevaluated the whole situation. Perhaps she and the doctor in Minnesota, who first diagnosed my nerve problem, were correct when they both said DO NOT RIDE THE BIKE. Even though I had no butt pain (yes, some did come later), there was no question that this recent cycling venture made my pubic/bladder area pain worse. Sure, I had demonstrated that I could ride a bicycle faster, but at what price? In the process of preparing this text, I realized I had made many stupid mistakes. With "20-20 hindsight" some of these should have been extremely obvious. Instead of solving problems, I was likely doing things to create more. The one unpardonable sin was drifting far afield from Dr. Antolak's ABSOLUTELY DO NOT DO instructions. I can provide complete assurance that they were followed during the first 15 months of treatment where results were spectacular (zero pain, no evidence of discomfort whatsoever in the butt or pubic/bladder area). During this period swimming was a prime source for me of aerobic exercise. I used a pull buoy to avoid the kick. Sometime after the first year of treatment, however, and I can not accurately pinpoint the time frame, I abandoned the swim and moved on to other gym exercise. I could not tell one exactly what or tell someone how much effort I put into it. Problems with my back seemed to dominate the picture and somehow I ignored several MUST AVOID parameters needed to properly control my pudendal neuropathy. For one reason or another leg presses, the glute machine, the elliptical trainer, hip abduction exercises and ultimately cycling did creep into my overall conditioning program from the second to fifth years. I should have known better and offer my sincere apology to Dr. Antolak, who was totally looking out for my interests. He has spent a lifetime researching the pudendal nerve and treating people with pudendal neuropathy. I have always learned best through the School of Hard Knocks. In this case I learned that the patient must adhere to all of the DO-NOT-Dos outlined if he expects to maximize nerve health.

At the end of the fifth year, I recognized that I must revamp my exercise program immediately if I wanted to avoid further damage to my pudendal nerve. I had no idea at this point how much of the damage already done was permanent and how much might be reversible. My revised exercise program is described in Table 4.2. The program shown is generally consistent with Dr. Antolak's long list of DO-NOT-DOs.

The Sixth Year (2012)

As the sixth year began, I was hopeful that my pudendal nerve and pubic/bladder area pain symptoms (Chapter 5) would turn more positive. I was extremely fortunate to see them do so by the middle of the first quarter in the Sixth Year. I had essentially no signs of pubic/bladder area pain and very few signs of discomfort in the rear end when I sat down for long periods of time. I have continued with the Gabapentin at the 1200 mg/day level, hopeful that sometime in the near future I can further reduce the level.

Very shortly after the end of the first quarter of The Sixth Year (April 2012), my wife and I returned from a four-week relaxation and golf vacation in Florida. I was feeling wonderful. No pain or discomfort whatsoever in the butt, (yes, not at any time during a 3000-mile journey by car or when sitting on the golf cart) or pain symptoms in the pubic/bladder area. I am very encouraged by the fact that I had essentially replicated the amazing zero butt pain/zero pain pubic/bladder area/very low NIH-CPSI values recorded after the first year of treatment by Dr. Antolak.

Current Health (April 2012)

My "recovery" from pudendal neuralgia, interstitial cystitis, and low back and knee pain described at the end of Chapter 3 has been for me

Table 4.2: Revamped exercise program for year six (2012).

Life Fitness® Treadmill Easy Workout 4-5 Times/wk. 35 min. with 5 min. Programmed Cool Down 2.0% Grade, 3.5 MPH, 1.90 miles **Results** Max. HR 115 Min. HR 95 (After 5 min. cool down)	**Life Fitness® Treadmill** Aerobic Workout 1 Times/wk. 35 min. with 5 min. Programmed Cool Down 3.5 % Grade, 3.7 MPH, 2.00 miles **Results** Max. HR 130 Min. HR 100 (After 5 min. cool down)
30 Min. No Kick Swim (w/Pull Buoy) 1 Time/wk. **Back Bridging** 14 minutes (4 min. on – 1 min. rest – 4 min. on – 1 min. rest – 4 min. on) See Figure 4.1a for "on" position 3 times/wk. **Five Planks** (45 sec. on/30 sec. rest) See Figure 4.1b for "on" position 2 times/wk. **40 lb. Forearm Bar** 2 sets/12 reps 2 times/wk.	**Life Fitness®** Biceps Curl and Triceps Extension 60 lb. 2 sets/12 reps/machine 2 times/wk. **Life Fitness® Lat Pulldown** 90 lbs. 3 sets/12 reps. 2 times/wk. **Gravitron/Stairmaster®** Dip/Pullup Machine 85 lb. Set 1 set 10 Dips and 1 set 10 Pullups 2 times/wk. **15 lb. Dumbbell** Overhead, each arm 1 set/12 reps. 2 times/wk.

NOTE: All leg exercises other than moderate walking have been eliminated. Most exercises are done on a near-empty stomach.

(a)

(b)

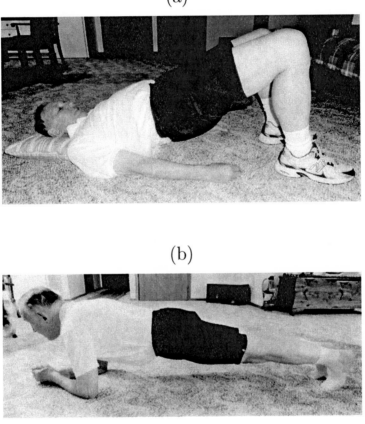

Figure 4.1: Stability Exercises. a) bridging exercise and b) plank exercise.

Resting heart rate	70
Blood pressure: systolic	110
Blood pressure: diastolic	70
Total cholesterol	161
HDL cholesterol	56
Triglycerides	74

Table 4.3: Some indicators to illustrate that my current diet and exercise program is functioning satisfactorily.

way beyond expectations. I can do all of the exercises cited in Table 4.2, without any discomfort whatsoever. Interstitial cystitis (discussed in Chapter 5) has rarely been a problem of concern. The only time I have noticed any difficulty is when I eat foods such as barbecue sauce or citrus and possibly a few others. Playing 18 holes of golf with zero back pain is a joy (the back pain issue has been addressed in Chapter 6). Today the right knee never aches and I can walk several miles per day without pain. For some time I have been taking three nutritional supplements daily with the bottom-line objective of maintaining or improving joint health (1500 mg glucosamine HCl, 1200 mg chondroitin sulfate and 2000 mg methylsulfonylmethane or MSM). I had been taking the glucosamine and chondroitin supplements prior to the knee problem, but not the MSM. If I had to make a guess as to the reason(s) for improvement in my knee, I would point to either the MSM or my new salmon-rich diet discussed in Chapter 8.

I regret the fact that in years 3 to 5 I did not show good pudendal nerve awareness. I realize it was wrong. In this book I am promoting nerve awareness and attempting to make certain that my thinking adheres to Dr. Antolak's DO-NOT-DOs. Table 4.3 below is a summary of current health markers which I believe should place me in the acceptable category. I am delighted with my current quality of life.

5

Interstitial Cystitis – The First New Problem – Diagnosis and Treatment

I must advise my readers upfront that I can look at this issue only with "20-20 hindsight." For some reason my "IC revelation" evolved about two years after my diagnosis of pudendal neuralgia as the reason for my butt pain. When I told Dr. Antolak of my interstitial cystitis experience, he told me he was not at all surprised (I thought IC was just a women's disease and something I would never acquire). He told me he believed that IC is really a component of pudendal neuralgia and actually represents a neurogenic inflammation of the bladder.

Symptoms

- Increased urination frequency. Bladder felt very irritated. Problems were worse at night.
- Periodic and seemingly increasing genital pain.
- General pelvic pain.

Diagnosis

My urologist, Dr. Tekchandani, made a confirming diagnosis via cystoscopy with hydrodistention under general anesthesia. Urine cultures showed no evidence of bacterial infection. Following surgery, Dr. Tekchandani showed me pictures of glomerations (pinpoints of bleeding) that are considered a hallmark of IC.

Initial Treatment

I was given a brochure which discussed in a general way my treatment options. Such included avoiding alcohol, spicy foods, chocolate, caffeine, citrus fruits, tomatoes and carbonated drinks if they worsened symptoms. For the most part, I avoided all of these foods as well as large doses of unbuffered vitamin C. I discovered from routine monitoring of urine PH that such would frequently drop to a level between 5.0 and 6.0. I wanted to keep it in the 6.5 to 7.5 range and was able to do so by better controlling my blend of acid and alkali forming foods. MSM – Methyl Sulfonyl Methane – was also helpful in this regard. I found that by paying closer attention to my diet and using 600 milligrams per day of Gabapentin, I could significantly reduce the IC pain.

Sudden Intensification of Pain

The time frame was a little more than two years after I had first seen Dr. Antolak regarding the pudendal nerve problems. I had just recently seen my urologist regarding new IC pain. She prescribed Pyridium, which really seemed to help. However, the pain continued to worsen. During one weekend the pain became severe, and by Sunday was horrendous. The story is summarized in Chapter 4, 2nd Year Assessment of My Pudendal Neuralgia Treatment – the Meals on Wheels adventure.

5. INTERSTITIAL CYSTITIS – THE FIRST NEW PROBLEM – DIAGNOSIS AND TREATMENT

For the greater part of the last three years, I have kept the Gabapentin level at 1200 mg/day. The final update on my IC status is given at the end of Chapter 4 in conjunction with my current health assessment.

6

Severe Low Back Pain –
The Second New Problem –
Diagnosis and Recovery

For the most part this problem really developed after the pudendal nerve and interstitial cystitis problems had been identified and
treatment initiated.

The Pain

I was struggling with the many ramifications of IC when I finally
realized that part of my pain problem must be related to the joints
in my lower back. Golfing was getting much more difficult. The
biggest problem was bending over to pick up the ball, clubs, and
flag. My initial approach was to see if chiropractic treatment would
help, but that proved ineffective. The next step was to engage a
doctor, Leslie Schutz, M.D., who specialized in rehabilitation. One
of her first steps was to order an MRI of the lumbar spine.

The Problem

The MRI showed that I have degenerative changes of the lumbar spine, most pronounced at the L3-4 level where there is disk space narrowing. It showed mild degenerative grade 1 spondylolisthesis of L3 on L4 (deformation of the architecture of the vertebrae due to wear and tear that erodes the facet joints between the bones) and borderline narrowing of the spinal canal. Mild degenerative narrowing of the neural foramina (nerve openings) was noted as well. (The above provides a good explanation for why, in the last few years of my bike racing career, I would always experience pain when training or racing on the bike with the back in a severely bent over position.)

The Treatment

The focus of Dr. Schutz's treatment was primarily one of physical therapy aimed primarily at strengthening and stabilizing core muscles in my back, hips, pelvis and abdomen. The program was designed specifically to use exercise machines at the Midland, MI Community Center. The basic program involved the use of hip abduction, glute, leg press, lat pulldown, seated row machines and eventually an elliptical trainer. "Back bridging" and "planks" were added as two stability exercises which I could do at home. Because of significant suprapubic pain, I abandoned all leg press activity in the third year following my first pudendal nerve office visit. I continued all other exercise activity following initiation at progressively higher load levels, for three to four years.

With little doubt, this program improved the strength and stability of my back. Coupled with a new golf swing and a new diet (discussed in subsequent chapters) my back has felt better than it has in many years. No pain or discomfort whatsoever in playing 18 holes of golf.

HOWEVER, with the benefit of "20-20" hindsight, I have reached the firm conclusion that treatment rationale for the pudendal nerve

6. SEVERE LOW BACK PAIN – THE SECOND NEW PROBLEM – DIAGNOSIS AND RECOVERY

versus that for the back and spine is almost irreconcilable. I now recognize that I probably made a huge mistake by not initially sitting down with Dr. Schutz before starting treatment and discussing the extremely broad scope of Dr. Antolak's DO-NOT-DOs. On the other hand, at least subconsciously, I recognized that I had a conundrum on my hands. Tell everything to Dr. Schutz and I almost certainly would get the response that she had no way to help me which would leave me with no way to get relief from horrendous back pain ... or tell her nothing and take the chance that if I did not literally follow every one of the DO-NOT-DOs [with the exception of the "planks" (and possibly the lat pulldown and extended "back bridging" exercise) mentioned above in the basic back therapy treatment program, all other exercise fall on this list] I would very likely further damage the nerve and inhibit the effectiveness of any treatment.

I chose the latter approach, won the back therapy battle but lost the battle to treat the nerve. The direction in which I must proceed is clear and has been outlined in Chapter 4. The final update on my low back pain status is given at the end of Chapter 4 in conjunction with my current health assessment.

7

A Simple Golf Swing Which is Easy on the Back

One day I was talking to a local golf pro and owner of a golf business in my neighborhood. I told him that I might have to give up the sport because of unforgiving low back pain whenever I played a round of golf. He asked me if I was familiar with the Moe Norman Natural Golf Swing[1], and I told him I was not. He said that the Moe Norman swing is truly different from the more conventional golf swing which vigorously rotates the back and body. Moe's swing involves minimal rotation and stress on the back. After listening to him tell about local golfers, with back problems similar to mine, who were able to successfully implement Moe Norman's swing, I knew I had to search for more detail. I needed to understand the specific details of Moe's swing and find out how I could make such work for me.

Wikipedia, the free encyclopedia, provides some good background information on Moe Norman [7]. Moe was a Canadian professional golfer (born 1929, died 2004). From that source we read "His accuracy, his ability to hit shot after shot perfectly straight, gave him

---

[1]The author obtained information on swing mechanics from the Natural Golf Corporation: http://moenormangolfacademy.org, and the the Graves Golf Academy (Oklahoma City, OK, http://moenormangolf.com).

the nickname 'pipeline Moe' ... Norman's skills as a ball striker are legendary. Sam Snead, himself one of the all-time greatest golfers, once described Norman as the greatest striker of the ball. In January 2005, Tiger Woods, the biggest golf star of the modern era, told Golf Digest's Jaime Diaz that only two golfers in history have 'owned their swings': Moe Norman and Ben Hogan. Stated Woods, 'I want to own mine.'"

Modifying my clubs to make them adaptable to Moe Norman Natural Golf was very simple. The golf pro referenced above replaced my grips with larger ones which he said were critical to making my new swing work properly. With Moe's swing the club is held with a palm rather than a finger grip.

Natural Golf is based on the science of a single plane swing. Unlike most golfers, one starts with arms and club shaft on the same plane at setup. The arms and club are maintained in this plane as the golfer proceeds through the backswing and then the downswing. Properly executed, this swing avoids most of the timing/body coordination requirements associated with the more conventional golf swing in which arms and club start out on different planes.

Benefits of Moe Norman's Swing

Fewer moving parts from setup to impact, better shot accuracy and consistency, good for amateurs – less coordination of body rotation and arm movements needed, easier on back.

Drawback of Moe Norman's Swing

Lack of distance and shot flexibility for the highly trained and talented golfer.

8

Why I Went to a Salmon Rich Diet

Because of inflammation associated with pudendal neuropathy, interstitial cystitis and low back pain, I was motivated to look at diet. Could a modification possibly reduce inflammation or provide other significant health benefits? When browsing the literature, I found that both Omega 3 and Omega 6 fatty acids are needed in the diet. Omega 3's were reported to function in an anti-inflammatory manner, whereas Omega 6's actually promote inflammation. How should I proceed to increase the level of Omega 3's in my diet?

After browsing many, many articles, I realized that everyone was really telling one story. Our basic diet is different from that of our forefathers, and today because of such contains a much lower level of Omega 3 fatty acids than is required for significant health benefits. I relied on the Gale Encyclopedia of Medicine [3] for help. This encyclopedia addresses the topic of Omega 3 Fatty Acids in a comprehensive, easy-to-understand three-page report. Topics include potential health benefits of fatty acids, recommended dosage, safety, precautions and other issues. For example, Gale states in their review that the American Heart Association indicates that research has shown that Omega 3 fatty acids:

- decrease the risk of arrhythmias, which can lead to sudden cardiac death
- decrease triglyceride levels
- decrease the growth rate of atherosclerotic plaque
- lower blood pressure slightly

I have targeted for my diet three to four servings per week salmon (3 to 4 oz. serving size) for Omega 3 health benefit. I believe the potential heart benefits alone justify such. Whether or not the anti-inflammatory properties of Omega 3's have significant impact on my pudendal nerve, IC or low back pain has not been established and may never be known.

9

Lessons Learned About the Use of Hyaluronic Acid For Better Skin, Joint and Eye Health

I have included this chapter in the text because I believed there was a reasonable chance that the use of an oral hyaluronic acid supplement might significantly improve my skin, joint and eye health. I even speculated that there was a chance that oral HA might help better cushion the pudendal nerve. After reading the book by Bill Sardi, *How to Live 100 Years Without Growing Old/Hyaluronic Acid: Nature's Healing Agent* [4], I was enthusiastic about all possibilities and wanted to evaluate the oral product myself. For reasons described below, I was unable to do so.

Lessons learned really turned out to be a tale of two stories.

The First Story

In the early part of 2011 I asked my personal physician, Dr. Malarz, if he could provide me with a hyaluronic acid based product to treat my face and neck. Much of the skin was sagging and had lost elasticity. There were many age spots, probably resulting from extensive sun exposure. There was residual damage left over from prior chemical peels, from treatment of several basal cell skin cancers and from childhood acne. To put it simply, my face was a mess. Dr. Malarz gave me a prescription for Bionect® gel[1] (as an 0.2% hyaluronic acid sodium salt) for topical application. Although the treatment process was slow, I could tell after two or three months use that it was being very effective. After about nine months of topical application, about 75% or more of the age spots had disappeared, my face was fuller, particularly in the cheeks, and it had developed significantly more elasticity. Skin was smooth as silk. I was delighted.

After about 15 months I terminated use of the product. My face was completely free of age spots and evidence of residual damage. Facial skin had good elasticity with almost zero sagging and negligible wrinkling.

The Second Story

Around mid-October 2011 I started what I hoped would be a long-term program to evaluate the efficacy of oral hyaluronic acid supplements. I was particularly interested in learning more about potential benefits to skin, joint and eye health (specifically glaucoma). Most of the literature I reviewed for these supplements indicated there were no significant side effects. I talked to a representative from the Neocell Corporation[2] who manufactured the product I was using and was told that there were no known side effects. The Neocell oral hyaluronic acid is the only one I have ever used.

When I first tried the Neocell product about four years ago, I felt distinct discomfort in the pubic/bladder area. Ability to urinate was reduced somewhat and I discontinued use of the product after about

---

[1]Bionect is manufactured by JSJ Pharmaceuticals, Inc., Charlston, SC (www.bionect.com).

[2]Neocell Corp., Newport Beach, CA (www.neocell.com).

two weeks. When I started my extended study, I started to use the product at the 50 mg/day level and then raised it to 100 mg/day (the suggested usage level) and kept it there for about two months.

During this time frame I had significant pain in the pubic/bladder area, particularly when lying down at night. The exact region seemed to correlate with the area where I had a TURP, which was performed 17 years ago. Again, while on the product I found it more difficult to urinate. I continued to use the product until the pain got so bad I had to reduce dosage to 50 mg/day.

After another two weeks at that level, I had to throw in the towel because of pain. To make absolutely certain that the problem lies with the oral HA supplement, I waited one more week and then took one 50 mg HA capsule. Same problem. In fact, it took 3 to 4 days to feel somewhat normal.

Conclusion: Oral Hyaluronic Acid Supplements are Contraindicated for me.

I believe that the primary source of my problem lies with the TURP surgery I had 17 years ago to address voiding problems and pubic/bladder area pain. The TURP surgery did not go well. I came out of such worse than when I went in. I believe the TURP surgery must have resulted in tissue scarring and possibly nerve damage. It has been reported in Bill Sardi's book that there are disorders where use of HA is contraindicated, and I believe this is clearly one of them. In an already scarred environment the more HA utilized, the more collagen generated resulting in a continued narrowing of the urinary tract. This explanation seems to fit perfectly with my experience.

10

Some Thoughts for Cyclists Wishing to Protect Butts and Body

Bicycling has the potential to seriously irritate or damage the nerves. Jim and Phil Wharton in the Whartons' Back Book address many of these concerns [6]. Common overuse injuries involve nerve compressions of the hand and forearm from pressure on the handlebar grip, nerve compression between the legs (i.e. the pudendal nerve) from sitting on a seat so hard that circulation is shut off; in the foot from wearing tight shoes, keeping too short a distance between the seat and pedals, and putting too much force down on the pedals for extended periods of time; pressure on the nerves of the cervical spine at the back of the neck from hyperextending the neck in holding the head up; lower backs trashed from many miles of training, keeping the back in flexion, bent over and stabilizing to hold the cyclist in an aerodynamic position.

General Considerations

- If pain develops in regions served by the pudendal nerve, it is best to discontinue cycling. Failure to do so could make the situation worse and cause improper functioning of the nerve. One should not delay diagnosis and treatment.
- Try to avoid constipation to reduce the possibility of stretching or damaging the pudendal nerve.

A Cyclist Checklist to Help Minimize Potential Problems

- ALWAYS WEAR A GOOD HELMET.
- Seat selection is critical – do not do extensive riding or training on a rock hard, narrow saddle which has essentially no support for the nerves and body parts which lie underneath. Choose a well-cushioned seat and one which helps diffuse the pressure.
- Use well-padded bike shorts.
- Vary your posture, periodically sit straight upright, take pressure off the back and neck; occasionally stand up on the pedals and take pressure off your butt.
- Wear properly sized, comfortable shoes and use well-padded gloves. Remove your hands from the grip one at a time and shake them to get blood flowing.
- Stay well hydrated. You will lose a lot of moisture on a hot, breezy day.
- Prepare for problems. A simple repair kit and cell phone may prove invaluable.
- Don't cycle in the dark without suitable lighting to appropriately identify yourself and the bike.
- Work to develop strong/flexible quadriceps muscles. They are crucial to powering the bike.

11

Some Concluding Thoughts and Lessons Learned

- The pudendal nerve originates in the pelvic region. The nerve is responsible for orgasm, urination and defecation. Its pathway may be tortuous among ligaments, muscles and other body structures, which if altered may damage the nerve.
- It is important for the bicycling and general community to have an awareness of the pudendal nerve and pudendal neuralgia. Good health and a pain-free life could depend on it. Such is a much larger issue than it might appear at first glance. I believe that 99+ percent of bicyclists have never heard of the pudendal nerve. Very few in the medical profession are well acquainted with the subject. Men and women have common symptoms for pudendal neuralgia. It does not seem to significantly impact one sex more than the other. It does not appear to be age related. The cyclist can be particularly vulnerable to pudendal neuralgia. Prolonged sitting often with poorly padded cycling shorts on hard, narrow poorly designed and positioned saddles, coupled with repetitive movement and hard thrusting of the legs may seriously compromise the health of the nerve. A major symptom of PN is pain when sitting, but genital pain is not uncommon. Individuals prone to pudendal neuralgia in

addition to cyclists may be those who had chronic constipation and prior pelvic surgery (I experienced both of these), frequent infections, a hard fall, difficult childbirth or actual entrapment, each of which could remodel the nerve. The prevalence of pudendal neuralgia in this country appears to be unknown.

- The pain level associated with pudendal neuralgia should not be underestimated. My Meals on Wheels adventure described in the text provides a good example of the horrendous pain which can be associated with pudendal neuralgia. In this case, I had terrible pain in the entire pelvic area including genitals and "butt" (pain front and rear). Very fortunately I had developed pudendal nerve awareness and found the proper way to proceed. I learned from this experience, however, that it would be very easy for individuals truly having undiagnosed pudendal neuralgia to become suicidal (as some have). Before my first visit to Dr. Antolak could be scheduled, my wife had to drive me to the local emergency room because of excruciating pain in the "butt." I was given morphine. That was somewhat ineffective. After I told them that I was absolutely convinced that my pain related to the pudendal nerve, they gave me new, much more effective nerve medication. Lesson learned – it is critical to choose the correct medication for pain control. Such medications have very wide variations in effectiveness.

- It is very common to have injuries to the pudendal nerve misdiagnosed. In many cases such have gone undiagnosed for years. Part of the problem relates to the complex nature of the subject and part to the fact that a very limited number of people in the medical profession are trained to address such issues. My pudendal neuralgia was misdiagnosed five times by five different doctors as chronic non-bacterial prostatitis. Penny Allen wrote that Ken Renney, M.D., in his younger years was "an avid cyclist with severe genital pain and a diagnosis of chronic prostatitis who saw more than 60 urologists to no avail."[2] Dr. Renney went to France for treatment of PNE (entrapment of the pudendal nerve) by anatomist and surgeon, Prof. Robert, who wrote the first article about PNE syndrome and treatment. [Dr. Renney founded the center at Memorial Herman Fort Bend Hospital, Houston, where PNE is treated.]

- It could prove helpful for the reader to remember one's telltale symptom for pudendal neuralgia – the pain is aggravated by sitting and reduced to some degree by standing, recumbent or sitting on a toilet. Pain in the genitals may also occur.

- Recognizing the symptoms of potential nerve damage is very important. Try not to continue activity which might further the damage. Once the damage reaches a certain point, it may become irreversible.

- My friend Kris in Belgium was an avid cyclist and runner who developed pudendal neuralgia at age 40. Unfortunately it took nearly three years for his problems to be characterized as such. His pudendal nerve was entrapped and his life turned completely upside down. He could not sit, a basic requirement for his job in Information Technology. His story helps illustrate that in Europe, as in the United States, there is limited medical expertise to adequately address and treat such issues. Kris is certain that he got PNE from cycling and he recommends to other bicyclists padded cycling shorts (Kris never used them) and a softer seat if one exists before you feel any pain. [See my text for more detail on Kris.]

- Treatment rationale to address pudendal nerve injury is almost irreconcilable with that normally prescribed for treatment of the back and spine. In cases such as mine, this presents a real conundrum. After successful stabilization of my back, I should never have continued to drift so far afield from my pudendal nerve doctor's DO-NOT-DO instructions, because in so doing I risked permanent damage to the nerve. I did some foolish things in this regard.

- My rehabilitation therapy doctor for the back and spine provided two wonderful exercises. They were the back bridging and plank exercises described in Chapter 4, Table 4.2 and Figure 4.1. Without the back bridging exercise, I believe there would be no chance of my playing golf and certainly not with zero pain. These exercises should also be very effective for cyclists as well as golfers who experience significant low back pain.

- My recovery is considered as complete as possible. The quality of life has returned. I can continue striving to make pars and birdies on the golf course. No, I cannot enjoy my first passion, bicycling and bicycle racing. Heart and lipid checks have shown that the diet and exercise programs described in the text have continued to keep my general health assessment at the satisfactory or above level.

- A primary objective in writing this book is to point out to the reader that there is hope for treating pelvic pain for which no definitive cause has yet been established. Such could be a nerve problem and relate specifically to the pudendal nerve, particularly if the pain occurs in the buttocks when sitting. Nerve medications may be very effective for pain control. I can tell the reader that for pudendal neuralgia cases such as mine, rapid progress with simple treatment can occur during the first year and such can be effectively measured.

- I was fortunate and very thankful to stumble by chance upon the pudendal nerve as the true cause of my problem, and to find a knowledgeable person who could refer me to a doctor who could help. In so doing, I may have avoided years of suffering. Do your research carefully!

- I hope from this text you have learned something that you did not know before about the pudendal nerve. Go out and enjoy cycling. It is a healthy sport. Build a passion for it. I would love to be riding and racing with all you 35 and 40 year olds, but it cannot be. When exploring country roads near farm houses, be careful. You may alert a rooster hidden in a roadside gulley wanting to cross the road right in front of you. Watch out for him. I did not.

Bibliography

[1] Penny Allen. Data show slow progress for surgical treatment of PNE. *Urology Times*, 33(2):18–20, February 2005.

[2] Penny Allen. Pudendal nerve entrapment may be mistaken for IC, CPPS. *Urology Times*, 33(2):17, February 2005.

[3] Laurie J. Fundukian, editor. *The Gale Encyclopedia of Medicine*. Gale, 4 edition, June 2011.

[4] Bill Sardi. *How to Live 100 Years Without Growing Old*. Here and Now Books, 2002.

[5] Donald Venes, editor. *Taber's Cyclopedic Medical Dictionary, 21st Edition*. F.A. Davis Company, 21 edition, February 2009.

[6] Jim Wharton and Phil Wharton. *The Wharton's Back Book*. Rodale Books, August 2003.

[7] Wikipedia contributors. Moe norman. http://en.wikipedia.org/wiki/Moe_Norman, April 2012.

[8] David Wise and Rodney Anderson. *A Headache in the Pelvis, a New Expanded 6th Edition: A New Understanding and Treatment for Chronic Pelvic Pain Syndromes*. National Center for Pelvic Pain Research, 5 edition, February 2011.

CPSIA information can be obtained at www.ICGtesting.com
Printed in the USA
BVOW082100241012

303835BV00002B/95/P

9 781477 216408